Julian L. Gallegos
West Lafayette, IN 47906
Jlgallegos@freedombroshealth.com

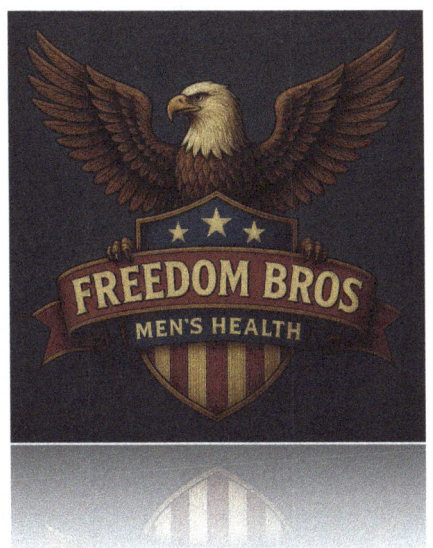

© **Freedom Bros. Men's Health, LLC**

Dedication

To my wife and son, you are my greatest blessings. Your support, sacrifice, and endless encouragement have sustained me through every season of this journey. Thank you for understanding the late nights, the long days, and the passion that pulled me into both the world of nursing and the fire service. Your love has been my anchor, my compass, and my light.

To every nurse I've worked alongside over the past 24 years— This book is for you. For the ones who kept showing up when the system didn't. For the ones who gave more than they had, and still felt unheard. For the ones carrying stories no one asks about. I see you. I hear you. And I wrote this because we deserve better not just for ourselves, but for those who will come after us.

And to the men and women of the fire service, thank you for welcoming me into your house, your rhythm, your culture. In the firehouse, I found the connection I had longed for throughout my nursing career. You gave me a seat at the table, a name among brothers and sisters, and a reason to believe in the power of showing up for one another again. You helped me rediscover purpose, not in policy but in people.

This book is born of love, written in gratitude, and offered in hope, that we might build a profession and a world where no one stands alone.

Prologue ....

Chapter 1 : Welcome to the Firehouse 1

Chapter 2 : The Brotherhood is Built, Not Assigned.....6

Chapter 3 : Brotherhood Is Inclusive, Not Exclusive ...12

Chapter 4 : Who Answers the Alarm? 18

Chapter 5 : Accountability at the Fire Scene..............23

Chapter 6 : Everyone Has a Role on the Rig...............29

Chapter 7 : Checking Your Gear 35

Chapter 8 : Kitchen Table Leadership 41

Chapter 9 : Honor the Sacrifice 47

Chapter 10 : The Call We All Heard 54

Chapter 11 : Lighting the Next Torch 60

Chapter 12 : A Profession Worth Saving 67

Epilogue: The Bell Tolls Once More 73

Workbook 77

Prologue

> *"I'd give it all up - every degree, every title, every accolade - just to be a firefighter."*

People look at me strangely when I say that. After all, I've been a nurse for over 24 years. I hold multiple degrees, certifications, leadership titles, and fellowships. On paper, I've built a successful career, one that's brought me to national stages, classrooms, and professional boardrooms. But behind every credential and honor is a truth I haven't always had the words to express: in all my years in nursing, I never truly felt like I belonged.

Not the way I did the moment I stepped into the firehouse.

When I joined as a volunteer firefighter, I wasn't chasing adrenaline or adding another title. I was searching, desperately for connection, which I didn't know, yet I found it. In the simplest, most profound ways: through shared meals, training shoulder to shoulder, laughs after calls, and the unspoken understanding that no one ever runs into a fire alone.

For the first time in my professional life, I didn't feel like I had to earn my place with overwork or perfection. I didn't need to prove my worth with degrees or explain my value. I was seen. I was heard. I was trusted. And I trusted back.

That kind of belonging is what we're missing in nursing, and it's costing us dearly.

We talk about burnout like it's an individual failure, but the real crisis is disconnection. Nurses are leaving the profession not because they can't handle the work, but because they feel invisible doing it. We've built systems that reward endurance and sacrifice, but rarely invest in human connection. We've replaced community with committees, replaced shared struggle with sterile silence.

And yet, in the fire service, a profession that also runs on trauma, urgency, and life-or-death stakes, they've figured it out. They lean on each other. They lead with loyalty. They build brotherhood not through bloodlines or bravado, but through belonging.

This book isn't about firefighting. It's about how **WE** save nursing.

It's a call to leaders: to rebuild the profession from the inside out, not with more policies, but with more presence. Not with metrics, but with meaning. To stop asking nurses to tough it out alone and start asking: What would it look like to lead like a firehouse captain? To create a team that trusts, a culture that connects, and a profession that sees its people not as providers, but as a family?

For every nurse who's ever felt like an outsider in their own profession, for every leader searching for a new way forward, this book is for you.

And it begins with a bell.

Not the one that marks the end of a shift, but the one that sounds when a brother or sister is lost. In the fire service, that bell is sacred. It rings in honor, in grief, and in remembrance.

It says:

We see you. You mattered. You will not be forgotten.

- *What would nursing look like if we rang that bell for each other?*

- *What would change if we built not just a workforce but a brotherhood?*

Let's find out.

- Julian L. Gallegos, Volunteer Firefighter. Nurse.

Leader on a mission to bring the fire back to nursing.

"Nursing Laid the Foundation, Firefighting Illuminated the Rest."

Chapter 1: Welcome to the Firehouse

"You don't just walk into a firehouse. You're welcomed into it."

The first time I stepped into the firehouse as a volunteer, I expected to feel out of place. After all, I was the nurse. The outsider. The one with the long résumé and a history in academia, not the type people picture suiting up for a fire. I expected to be greeted with skepticism, maybe even indifference.

But what I found was something entirely different.

I was welcomed.

Not with a formal ceremony or orientation checklist, but with a nod, a handshake, and a place at the table. Within hours, I was rolling hoses, swapping stories, and learning the rhythms of life in the bay. It was loud, it was raw, it was real, and for the first time in my professional life, I felt like I was part of something.

That firehouse didn't just offer me a new role. It offered me a home.

The Firehouse as Home

In the fire service, the station is more than just a workplace. It's a sacred space. It's where firefighters cook together, sleep under the same roof, and gather after calls to process the weight of what they've seen. The firehouse is where trust is forged not through forced team-building activities, but through presence the kind that says: "I've got your back."

Every firefighter knows that what happens inside the house is what determines how well they function outside of it. The strength of the crew isn't built during the fire, it's built in the quiet moments in between.

Contrast that with many nursing units, classrooms, or boardrooms. Our environments are often transient, fractured, and transactional. Nurses pass each other like ships in the night, often too busy to connect. Academics rush from meeting to meeting, rarely pausing to check in on each other's well-being. Executives make decisions in isolation, disconnected from the emotional pulse of their teams.

We Build What We Value

Here's the hard truth: the spaces we create reflect the values we uphold.

If we design systems that prioritize productivity over people, we shouldn't be surprised when our teams feel expendable. If we invest in policies but not in culture, we'll continue to lose talented professionals not to failure but to emptiness.

The fire service teaches us that culture is not an accident. It's intentional. It's maintained through ritual, storytelling, and shared vulnerability. It's sustained through leadership that shows up not just when something's wrong, but every day, in ordinary moments.

And it starts with welcoming people into the house, not just the profession.

Belonging Is a Leadership Responsibility

As nurse leaders, whether in academia, health systems, policy, or research, we cannot afford to treat belonging as a soft skill or an afterthought. Belonging is a strategic imperative. It is the foundation for resilience, innovation, collaboration, and retention.

Ask yourself:

- *Do your teams feel like they're working with each other or simply around each other?*

- *Do new members feel like they've joined a family or entered a trial period?*

- *Do your spaces physical and emotional communicate: "You belong here"?*

If not, it's time to rebuild the house.

Not with bricks, but with presence. Not with policies, but with people. Not with mandates, but with meaning.

The Kitchen Table Test

In every firehouse, there's a kitchen table. It's not fancy. Often scratched, stained, and worn. But it's the heart of the house. It's where stories are told, where trust is built, and where the team becomes more than a crew; it becomes a family.

What is the "kitchen table" in your organization?

Where do your people gather to be human?

If you can't name it, build it.

Leadership isn't just about strategy. It's about space. About creating an environment where people feel safe enough to care, courageous enough to speak, and seen enough to stay.

That's what the firehouse has taught me. And that's the leadership nursing desperately needs.

Welcome to the house. Let's make sure no one stands outside it again.

Leadership Flashpoint: Reflection Prompts

1. *Where in your current leadership environment do people naturally gather, and are those spaces inclusive?*

2. *How have you (intentionally or unintentionally) contributed to isolation or disconnection on your team?*

3. *What's one tradition, ritual, or informal space you can establish to build connection this month?*

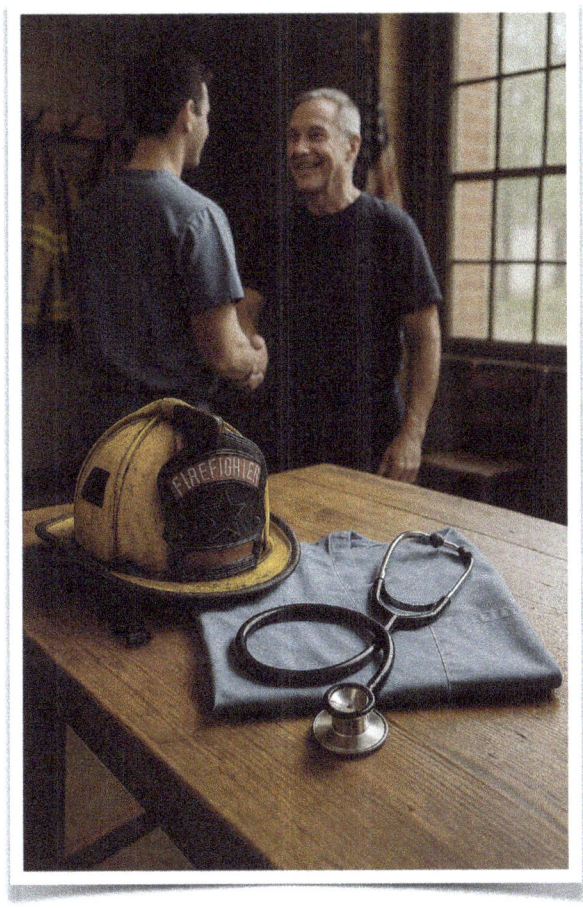

Chapter 2 : The Brotherhood is Built, Not Assigned

"You don't get the brotherhood just by showing up. You earn it, by showing up for each other."

In the fire service, they don't hand you a sense of belonging with your turnout gear. You don't get called "brother" or "sister" on day one. It's not a title; it's a relationship, forged in the heat of shared experience and the quiet consistency of being there when it counts.

That's what makes it powerful.

I learned this quickly after joining the fire service. No one made a big deal about my arrival. There was no speech, no banner. But there was a clear expectation: Pull your weight. Be accountable. And watch out for your crew. Over time, as we trained, ran calls, and ate together, something shifted. They didn't just accept me; they trusted me.

That trust didn't come from my degrees or my background. It came from my actions. From listening, showing up, asking questions, and having their backs. That's how brotherhood is built. Slowly. Intentionally. Through presence, humility, and consistency.

And that's precisely what nursing leadership often overlooks.

Assigned Teams vs. Built Relationships

In nursing, especially in large organizations, academic institutions, and bureaucratic systems, teams are often assigned rather than built. We're grouped by title, function, or department. We're expected to work together effectively, even when we've barely spoken. The assumption is that professionalism alone will bind us.

But it doesn't.

Because professionalism without human connection is just performance.

A fire crew wouldn't dare run into a burning structure with someone they've never trained with. Yet in nursing, we ask teams to tackle moral distress, crises, and life-or-death situations without the benefit of trust, familiarity, or psychological safety.

That's not just a leadership oversight, **it's a leadership failure**.

Trust is the Currency of High-Performing Teams

One of the most common phrases you'll hear in the fire service is: "I'd trust that person with my life." It's not said lightly. It means the person has proven, again and again, that they show up, do their job, and watch out for their crew.

Nursing must reclaim this level of trust.

Too often, we substitute procedure for partnership. We implement tools like SBAR, huddles, and standardized handoffs, thinking they're enough. But without relational trust, these tools are just templates.

High-performing teams aren't built on checklists, they're built on connection.

Leadership in nursing must move beyond structural organization and toward relational integration. That means creating time, space, and culture for team members to get to know each other as people, not just as roles.

Ask yourself:

- *Does your team trust each other enough to be vulnerable?*

- *Can they admit when they're struggling, without fear of judgment?*

- *Do they step in for one another, not because it's expected but because it's who they are?*

> If not, it's time to stop managing teams and start building brotherhood.

The Myth of the Lone Nurse

There's a damaging myth in nursing: the heroic lone nurse who powers through every shift, never asks for help, and bears the emotional burden of others without breaking.

This myth is killing us.

It isolates. It breeds shame. It discourages collaboration. And it flies in the face of everything we know about human resilience and performance.

The fire service doesn't operate this way. No one goes in alone. Ever. Not into a structure fire, not into a rescue. Why? Because they know that survival depends on teamwork, trust, and coordination.

So why do we continue to romanticize the isolated nurse hero?

Leadership must dismantle the culture of silent suffering and replace it with collective responsibility. Not just for the work, but for each other.

Building Brotherhood in Nursing: A Leadership Imperative

Let me be clear: "brotherhood" in this book doesn't refer to gender or exclusivity. It's about a deep, enduring sense of mutual commitment and belonging. Brotherhood is knowing someone has your back before you ask. It's trusting that no one will let you fall through the cracks. It's feeling seen not just for your output, but for your humanity.

That kind of culture doesn't happen by chance.

It is built through mentorship, honest conversations, shared purpose, and leadership that models vulnerability, not perfection.

Leadership Reflection:

- *Are you creating an environment where brotherhood can grow?*

- *Or one where people feel disposable?*

Because here's the truth:

Connection isn't a perk. It's not a "nice to have." It is the oxygen that keeps the fire of our profession alive.

Without it, burnout wins.

With it, we build something that endures, not just a workforce, but a family.

Leadership Flashpoint: Reflection Prompts

1. *What are you doing, intentionally, to build relational trust on your team?*

2. *When was the last time you asked someone how they're really doing and stayed to listen?*

3. *What rituals, spaces, or routines could you introduce to shift your team from assigned roles to shared brotherhood?*

Voices from the Fire Service:

"I don't need you to be the strongest or the smartest. I need to know you'll show up for me when it counts. That's what makes you part of this crew."
- Captain, Volunteer Fire Department

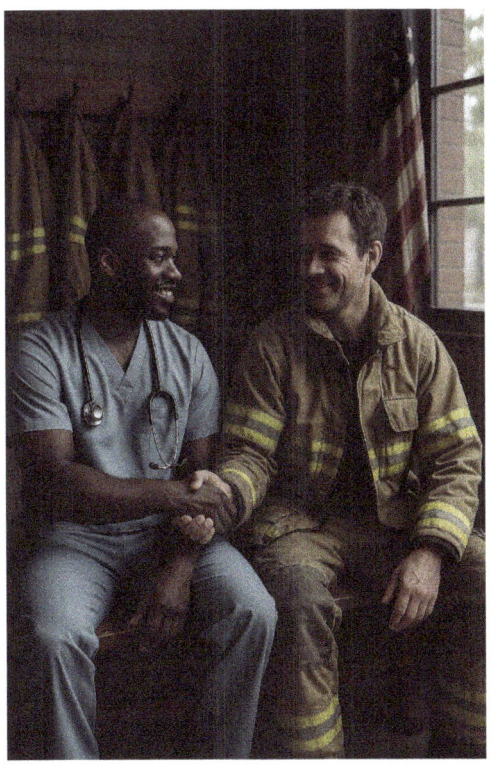

Chapter 3 : Brotherhood Is Inclusive, Not Exclusive

"Brotherhood isn't about sameness. It's about solidarity."

Walk into most firehouses today and you'll still hear the word brotherhood used with reverence. It doesn't mean you share a last name, background, or belief system. It means you show up for each other, no matter what. It means that in moments of danger, difference fades and unity steps forward. We fight together. We fall together. We rise together.

But even in the fire service, where brotherhood is a badge of honor, the culture had to evolve. It had to become more open, more aware, and more intentional about who got a seat at the table and who didn't.

Nursing finds itself at a similar crossroads.

We speak about community and caring. We preach inclusion and advocacy. Yet too often, we build silos within our own profession:

- Men in nursing feel like outsiders in a historically female profession.

- Nurses of color are expected to conform to white norms of professionalism.

- LGBTQIA+ nurses must weigh safety against authenticity.

- Nurses from lower socioeconomic backgrounds are often excluded from advancement.

- And those who don't fit the dominant culture quietly question whether they ever truly belonged.

> Brotherhood, true brotherhood, isn't just about connection.
>
> It's about making space.
>
> It's about seeing difference and still saying: You are one of us.

Brotherhood Is a Mindset, Not a Demographic

> Some bristle at the word brotherhood. They see it as gendered, outdated, and exclusive.

But in this book, brotherhood is a metaphor, one drawn from the fire service that transcends gender and race. It's about deep, unshakable connection rooted in loyalty, trust, and shared purpose. It's about being part of something that protects you, even when you're not the same.

So what does that mean for nursing?

It means creating cultures where no one has to leave their identity at the door in order to belong. It means ensuring our communities are not just diverse in appearance, but inclusive in power, voice, and validation.

It means saying:

- "You don't have to assimilate to be accepted."

- "You are not here on sufferance, you are essential."

- "We don't just tolerate you, we need you."

Nursing must stop gatekeeping belonging.

The Price of Exclusion

Let's be honest: exclusion doesn't always show up in open discrimination. More often, it's subtle. It shows up in the offhand comment. The missed invitation. The biased evaluation. The all-white leadership team. The unwillingness to pronounce someone's name correctly.
Exclusion whispers: You're not one of us.
And eventually, that whisper becomes internalized and people leave.

Leaders, this is on us.

When a profession as diverse as nursing still struggles to make all its members feel seen, safe, and supported, we are not facing a diversity issue; we are facing a leadership issue.

Because inclusion doesn't happen by default. It happens by design.

And in spaces where connection is the foundation of resilience, healing, and trust, exclusion is not just morally wrong; it's professionally devastating.

Brotherhood Demands Intentional Inclusion

In the fire service, the crew doesn't just "happen"; it's built. Senior firefighters take time to mentor rookies. Officers notice when someone is being left out. There are systems for onboarding, for checking in, for team cohesion.

That's intentional.

Nursing needs the same approach. We can't assume belonging happens organically. We must engineer it.

Ask yourself:

- Do new nurses from underrepresented backgrounds have mentors who understand their journey?

- Are diverse voices represented in leadership, not just in attendance, but in influence?

- Do we address micro-aggressions or bury them in silence?

Building inclusive brotherhood means having hard conversations, listening more than speaking, and letting go of the idea that culture should always feel comfortable for you.

Growth is uncomfortable.

Inclusion is humbling.

But both are necessary.

Inclusion is the Future of Connection

You cannot build real connection without inclusion.

It's not enough to say, "Everyone is welcome."
You must show it. Prove it. Live it.

That means:

- Creating space for nurses to bring their whole selves to the profession.

- Amplifying the stories of those too often left out of the narrative.

- Understanding that equity isn't giving everyone the same thing, it's giving everyone what they need to succeed.

- And accepting that belonging is a feeling, not a policy.

Leadership isn't just about getting the job done. It's about cultivating a team where everyone can do their best work, safely and authentically.

Brotherhood doesn't mean we are the same. It means we stand together, especially when we're different.

Leadership Flashpoint: Reflection Prompts

4. Who in your team or organization might be feeling unseen or outside the circle of connection?

5. What systems, habits, or "norms" might unintentionally exclude people who don't fit the dominant culture?

6. How can you lead more intentionally to build a team where everyone feels they belong–not just the ones who look, think, or act like you?

Voices from the Fire Service:

"Brotherhood doesn't mean we're all the same. It means I'll run through the fire for you, no matter who you are–because we're in this together."
- Firefighter-Paramedic, Urban Station

Chapter 4 : Who Answers the Alarm?

"We all run toward the sound of the bell. But what matters most is who shows up and why."

The alarm doesn't discriminate. When it sounds in the firehouse, there's no time to ask whose job it is, who's feeling tired, or who's new to the team. Everyone moves. Everyone responds. Because lives depend on it.

The alarm doesn't discriminate. When it sounds in the firehouse, there's no time to ask whose job it is, who's feeling tired, or who's new to the team. Everyone moves. Everyone responds. Because lives depend on it.

But it's not just the urgency of the situation that gets people out of bed; it's trust in the crew and the unbreakable code that you never leave your brothers and sisters behind.

In nursing, we face alarms too. Sometimes they come in the form of actual codes. More often, they're quieter: a colleague overwhelmed on a shift, a new educator unsure of their place, a student drowning in self-doubt, or a seasoned nurse teetering on the edge of burnout.

Yet how often do we answer those alarms?

How often do we even hear them?

The truth is, our profession is full of silent alarms, cries for help, belonging, mentorship, and meaning. But in our hyper-tasked, hyper-efficient systems, we've been trained to respond only to what's chartable, billable, or policy-driven.

Leadership, true leadership, requires that we tune back in.

The Call Is Personal

One of the most profound lessons I've learned in the fire service is this: Every call is personal. Whether it's a major accident or a cat in a tree, it matters to someone. And so it must matter to us.

When the alarm sounds, no one rolls their eyes or picks and chooses based on what they feel like doing that day. They answer because the mission comes first, and the crew comes with them.

That's a mindset we need to resurrect in nursing.

As leaders, we've allowed disconnection and overwork to desensitize us. We see turnover as a trend, not as trauma. We call burnout a statistic, not a signal. We wait until people leave to realize they were sounding the alarm for months.

What if, instead, we took every emotional alarm as seriously as a code blue? What if the call was personal again?

Who's Missing From the Rig?

Every firehouse has a roll call, a literal check of who's present before a call. If someone's missing, you notice. You ask. You follow up. Because you can't afford to fight the fire short-staffed or with uncertainty.

In nursing, we often move forward without doing a roll call, figuratively or literally. We don't check in on who's present mentally, emotionally, or spiritually. We assume everyone is fine until they're not. Until they resign. Until they break. Until they become "just another burnout story."

But here's the thing: burnout has a face. Disengagement has a name. And the missing from the rig are people we knew– colleagues, students, friends.

Leadership must commit to a culture of active presence– where we notice who's gone quiet, who's pulling away, who needs someone to ask, "Are you okay?" and mean it.

Because the ones who don't answer the alarm are often the ones we never truly showed up for in the first place.

The Burden of Unanswered Alarms

There's a weight that firefighters carry when they lose someone in a call. It stays with them not just as grief, but as reflection: Did we do everything we could? Were we there for them when it mattered?

Nursing carries a different weight– the burden of the unspoken, the unnoticed, the unfelt.

Leaders must confront this burden honestly. How many calls have we missed because we were too busy, too distracted, or too focused on output? How many nurses walked away from the profession because no one saw the signs?

Answering the alarm in nursing isn't about always having solutions. It's about showing up, consistently, intentionally, and with humility. It's about letting your team know:

You're not alone. I hear you. I'm with you.

Leadership in the Line of Fire

In the fire service, the officer on the truck doesn't bark orders from the back. They're on the front lines. They assess risk, make the hard calls, and stand shoulder to shoulder with their team.

Nursing leadership must do the same.

You can't lead connection from behind a desk. You can't build trust from a Zoom screen. You must be in the house, at the bedside, in the meeting, around the table–wherever the alarm sounds.

Because your presence as a leader is more powerful than any speech, policy, or strategic plan. It tells your team, "You matter. I hear the alarm too. And I'll answer it with you."

Leadership Flashpoint: Reflection Prompts

7. What alarms, literal or figurative, are you missing in your organization?

8. Who's become quiet, withdrawn, or invisible? When did you last check in?

9. How can you build a culture where emotional alarms are responded to with the same urgency as clinical ones?

Voices from the Fire Service:

"You don't have to be the one inside the fire to feel the heat. If your crew's in there, you're in it too because no one fights alone."
- Veteran Firefighter and EMT

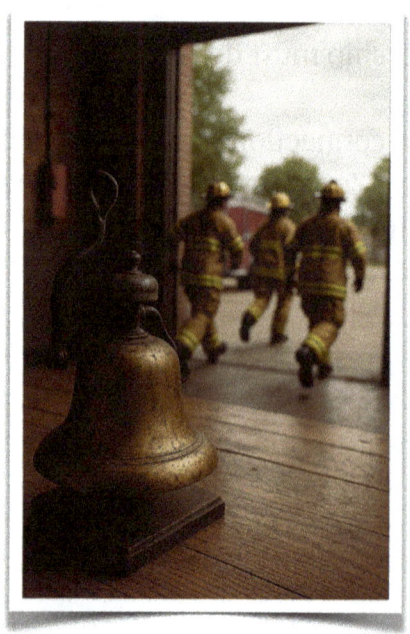

Chapter 5 : Accountability at the Fire Scene

"On the fireground, accountability isn't optional; it's survival."

In the fire service, when the call comes in and the crew arrives on the scene, everyone knows what to do. There is no confusion, no duplication, no hiding. Each firefighter has a role, clear, practiced, and trusted. The officer assumes command. The driver sets the pump. The interior team advances the hose. The ladder crew handles ventilation. The accountability officer tracks every single person entering and exiting the building.

- **No one freelances.**

- **No one disappears.**

- **No one works without being known.**

Because in a fire, chaos is waiting to kill you, and accountability is what keeps you alive.

Now think about healthcare. Think about nursing teams in crisis: a patient coding, a system failing, a unit short-staffed, a department under investigation. Does every person know their role? Is leadership clearly defined? Is trust present and visible?

Too often, the answer is no. Not because we lack competence, but because we lack clarity, consistency, and connection. In other words, we lack accountability culture.

Accountability Is Not About Blame; It's About Belonging

Let's be honest: in many nursing environments, "accountability" has become a dirty word. It's been weaponized to punish mistakes rather than promote growth. It's become synonymous with surveillance, correction, or disciplinary action.

But in the fire service, accountability is the opposite of punishment; it's protection. It means someone is keeping track of you because they care whether you come back alive. It means you're never left behind, never invisible, never an afterthought.

True accountability is an act of altruism.

It says, "I see you. I know what you're doing. And I'll make sure no one forgets to look for you if things go south."

Nursing leadership must reclaim this version of accountability, not as control, but as care.

Chain of Command = Chain of Trust

In the fireground, the chain of command isn't just about rank. It's about response. Every person knows who they report to, who's making the decisions, and who's responsible for their safety.

This clarity allows for rapid action and team cohesion in even the most dangerous environments. It removes ambiguity. It prevents the "too many captains, not enough crew" problem. And it reinforces psychological safety, because people know who to turn to when the heat rises– literally and figuratively.

In contrast, nursing often suffers from blurred lines of leadership. Leaders are absent or inaccessible. Middle managers are overburdened. Faculty lack mentoring from above. And staff nurses are expected to lead "from below" without the authority or support to do so.

In this vacuum, people flounder or, worse, disengage.

Leadership must restore a visible, trustworthy chain of command. Not just on org charts, but in practice. Nurses at every level should know:

- Who is leading me?

- Do I trust them to lead with integrity?

- Can I go to them without fear of retaliation or dismissal?

When those answers are unclear, disconnection sets in. But when they're solid, accountability becomes a shared value, not a top-down imposition.

Mutual Accountability Builds Brotherhood

Fire crews hold each other accountable every day, not just in emergencies. They check each other's gear. They remind each other to hydrate. They train together. They correct each other without humiliation, because their lives depend on it.

That level of mutual respect is rare in nursing.

Instead, we too often fall into horizontal violence, avoidance, or passive aggression. We see a mistake but don't speak up. We feel overwhelmed but don't ask for help. We watch someone struggle but stay silent because we've learned that accountability might lead to shame, not support.

Leaders must model mutual accountability:

- **Admit your own mistakes.**

- **Ask for feedback.**

- **Create environments where speaking up is a gift, not a risk.**

Because when people trust each other enough to correct each other with kindness, that's when real professional maturity emerges.

Debriefing: The Missing Ritual

Every major fire ends with a debrief. The team circles up and discusses what went well, what could have gone better, and what needs to change next time. No one is exempt. Everyone contributes. The goal is collective growth, not individual fault-finding.

This kind of structured reflection is desperately missing in nursing.

We rush from crisis to crisis, from semester to semester, from project to project, without pausing to ask, " What did we learn? How can we grow together?" Without debriefing, we miss the opportunity to transform accountability into learning.

Leaders must institutionalize reflective practices.

Whether it's a monthly team huddle, post-event reviews, or anonymous surveys, every group needs a rhythm of transparent, shared reflection.

That's how accountability moves from being reactive to being proactive and empowering.

Leadership Flashpoint: Reflection Prompts

10. *When was the last time you debriefed a major project, crisis, or failure with your team?*

11. Do the people you lead know exactly who they can turn to in a crisis, and do they trust that person?

12. Have you created a culture where giving and receiving feedback is normalized and non-punitive?

Voices from the Fire Service:

"When you walk into a burning building, you don't think about your ego. You think about your people. You do the job, and you watch each other's backs. That's what accountability means to us."
- Lieutenant, County Fire Department

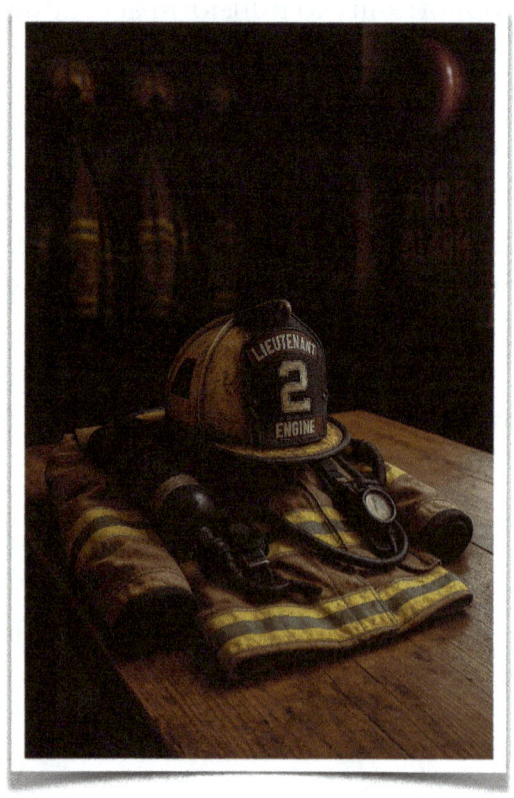

Chapter 6 : Everyone Has a Role on the Rig

"You don't have to do everything; you just have to do your job. And trust that your crew will do theirs."

There's something beautiful about the choreography of a fire scene. Without shouting or chaos, a dozen people move with purpose. The driver sets the pump. The nozzle team stretches the line. The officer establishes command. The ladder crew goes to the roof. The medic preps the stretcher. No one waits for permission. No one gets in someone else's way. And no one stands around unsure of what they're supposed to be doing.

Why? Because everyone knows their role and respects everyone else's.

That clarity saves lives.

And that respect builds trust.

Now imagine if healthcare functioned like that.

Imagine an academic team where the educator didn't micromanage the clinician, where the researcher didn't undervalue the educator, where administrators supported from behind rather than controlled from above. Imagine if each person, from nurse to dean, new grad to seasoned scholar, felt their contribution was understood, essential, and honored.

That's not fantasy. That's how it should be.

And leadership is responsible for making it happen.

The Power of Role Clarity

In the fire service, every member of the crew is cross-trained. But even with shared knowledge, they don't all do the same thing on the scene. The key to efficiency and survival is knowing whose job is whose, and trusting your team to do it.

In nursing, however, we often blur roles intentionally or not. Staff nurses are expected to act as case managers, social workers, and sometimes even security guards. Faculty are asked to teach, advise, research, serve, and somehow maintain a full clinical practice. Nurse leaders are pulled in so many directions, they struggle to lead at all.

The result is role dilution, which leads to role confusion, which leads to disconnection and resentment.

When people don't know what's expected of them or, worse, when they constantly do others' jobs out of necessity or dysfunction, they don't feel like valued members of a team. They feel like cogs in a broken machine.

Leadership must protect role clarity as a form of professional dignity.

That means:

- Defining expectations clearly and communicating them consistently.

- Respecting boundaries while promoting collaboration.

- Trusting others to perform their duties without micromanagement or judgment.

When everyone has a role on the rig and knows it, the team flows.

The Role of the Quiet Leader

Not everyone on a fire crew is the loudest, fastest, or most experienced. Some are quiet giants. The ones who check the air packs without being asked. The ones who double-check the rig before bed. The ones who say little but always show up.

In nursing, these people often go unnoticed. They don't seek the spotlight, but their impact is enormous. They're the culture carriers, the behind-the-scenes stabilizers, the emotional anchors of the team.

Leadership must develop the vision to see the quiet leaders, to recognize the contributions that aren't flashy but are foundational. If we only reward those who speak the loudest or submit the most, we miss out on the deep strength of those who simply do their job with heart.

Great crews are not made up of superstars. They're made up of consistent, dependable people who trust each other to show up and do the work together.

The Danger of Over-functioning

In a dysfunctional fireground, someone might try to do everything: pull hose, run command, ventilate the roof, and provide care. That person isn't a hero; they're a liability. Their over-functioning puts the entire team at risk.

Nursing is full of "over-functioners". Leaders who do instead of delegate. Educators who take on students' burdens rather than empower them. Nurses who pick up everyone's slack because they're afraid to speak up or set boundaries.

Over-functioning may look noble, but it's often rooted in fear: fear of failure, fear of letting others down, and fear that the team isn't trustworthy.

Leadership must break this cycle.

You can't build a healthy team if no one is allowed to rise. You can't cultivate trust if you're constantly doing it all yourself.

The fire service teaches this lesson clearly: Know your job. Do your job. Trust your crew to do theirs.

That's how teams grow. That's how leaders develop. That's how professions thrive.

Building Role Identity in Nursing

To build strong nursing teams across practice, academia, and leadership, we must help each person develop a clear, confident professional identity. Not just, "What is your title?" but:

- What is your purpose?

- What is your lane?

- Where are you most trusted, effective, and alive in your work?

Leaders should ask and help answer these questions for their teams regularly. Role clarity isn't static; it evolves. But that evolution must be guided, not assumed.

If someone on your team can't tell you what their role is or if they tell you they wear too many hats to count, that's a leadership failure, not a personal one.

Let's stop handing out hats and start helping people wear the right one proudly and with purpose.

Leadership Flashpoint: Reflection Prompts

1. Do your team members have clarity about their roles, and are those roles aligned with their strengths and passions?

2. Are you over-functioning in areas where others should be empowered to lead?

3. When was the last time you celebrated someone for doing their quiet, consistent, vital role well?

Voices from the Fire Service:

"I don't need you to do my job—I need you to do yours. Because if we all do our jobs, no one gets left behind."
- Fire Captain, Midwestern Volunteer Department

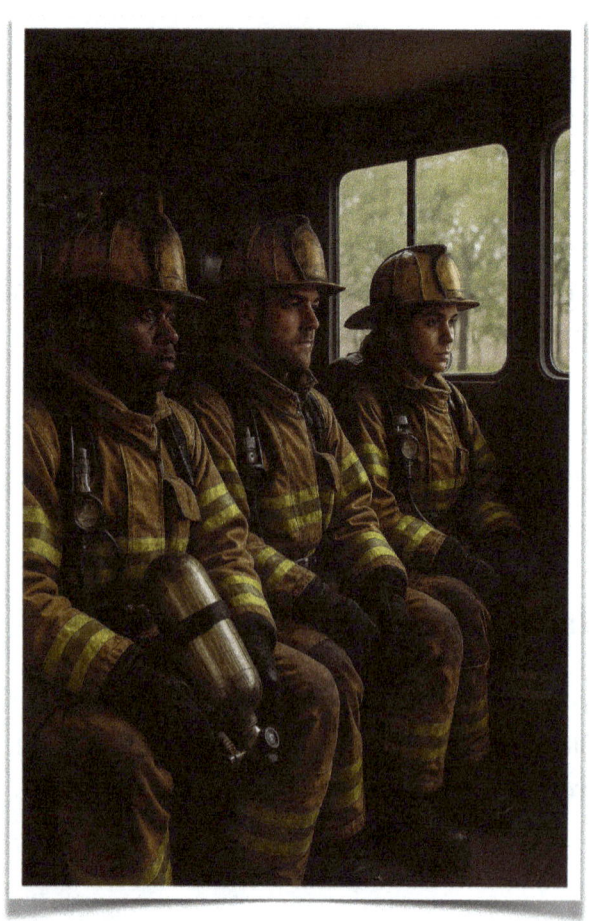

34

Chapter 7 : Checking Your Gear

"You don't enter the fireground with unchecked gear. Why do we enter our workday with unchecked minds?"

In the fire service, gear checks are sacred. Before every shift, firefighters inspect every piece of their equipment: helmets, air packs, turnout gear, gloves, boots. They clean it, adjust it, test it. Not because someone told them to, but because their life depends on it. And so does the life of the person next to them.

It's routine. It's expected. It's ingrained.

Now consider the nursing profession.

How many nurses, educators, leaders, or executives check their emotional gear before starting their day? How often do we ask ourselves:

- Am I mentally ready for what I'm about to face?

- Do I have the emotional capacity to lead, to teach, to care?

- Am I carrying unprocessed trauma from yesterday into today?

The answer, far too often, is: I don't have time to ask.

That's a leadership crisis. Because unlike malfunctioning gear, which we can see, touch, and replace, unseen emotional strain festers in silence. And when ignored, it becomes exhaustion, burnout, withdrawal, resentment, and ultimately, attrition.

In fire, gear is checked to save lives.

In nursing, emotional gear must be checked to save ourselves.

Emotional Readiness Is Professional Readiness

The fire service doesn't just train for technical skill; they prepare their minds. They run drills. They walk through worst-case scenarios. They practice staying calm under pressure. They debrief after every call, not just for outcomes, but for impact.

This isn't just tactical, it's emotional hygiene. It keeps the team healthy.

In nursing, we often skip this step. We treat emotional readiness like a luxury. We reward stoicism and call it strength. We dismiss check-ins and call them "soft skills." But the truth is, ignoring the emotional gear check is why so many nurses crash later.

Leadership must change the narrative.

You cannot lead with clarity if your mental fog goes unchecked.

You cannot sustain a profession that denies its people the time to breathe.

We need a cultural shift from gear up and go to check your gear and grow.

Leaders Set the Tone for Psychological Safety

In a firehouse, the officer sets the tone for every shift. If they rush the gear check, the crew rushes. If they skip debrief, others will too. If they model composure, accountability, and care, the crew follows.

Nursing leadership must do the same.

When leaders show up frazzled, disengaged, or emotionally unavailable, the team feels it. People begin to mask, to shrink, to cope in isolation. But when leaders lead with presence, humility, and openness, they give others permission to do the same.

Psychological safety isn't built by HR departments or wellness apps. It's built by leaders who:

- Ask, "How are you, really?"and wait for the answer.

- Model vulnerability without weakness.

- Normalize rest and recovery without shame.

- Debrief without blame.

A psychologically safe team doesn't just feel better–they perform better, support each other more, and stay longer.

The Silent Weight of the Unchecked

In the fire service, if you forget to check your air tank or flashlight, you risk getting trapped in darkness or smoke. The consequences are immediate and often fatal.

In nursing, the consequences of emotional neglect are slower, but just as dangerous. When nurses and leaders alike suppress their fatigue, trauma, and moral distress, it doesn't disappear. It embeds itself in the culture. It spills out in snide remarks, passive resistance, missed opportunities, and emotional disengagement.

Unchecked pain becomes unspoken pain.

Unspoken pain becomes normalized pain.

And normalized pain becomes culture.

Leadership must break this cycle. And it starts with modeling the daily emotional gear check.

Ask yourself:

- What am I carrying from yesterday that I need to name?

- Who do I need to connect with today?

- What do I need to release so I can lead with clarity?

Then teach your team to do the same.

Make it a ritual. Build it into meetings. Normalize it in conversation.

Because when you check your gear, you're not just preparing to do the job; you're preparing to do it well, with presence and purpose.

The Gear of Connection

Firefighters don't just check personal gear. They check the truck. They check each other. They ask if everyone is ready.

That's what makes it a crew, not just individuals doing a job.

Nursing must reclaim this team readiness model. Before a shift. Before a class. Before a big decision.

Leaders can ask:

- Are we ready?

- Does anyone need support before we begin?

- What are we carrying, and how can we carry it better– together?

The check-in doesn't need to be long. But it needs to be real.

When people feel seen before the work starts, they bring their best. When they feel invisible, they protect themselves, and the team loses something irreplaceable.

Leadership Flashpoint: Reflection Prompts

4. What personal check-ins or rituals do you practice to assess your own emotional readiness?

5. How do you create space for your team to speak up if they are emotionally or mentally unwell?

6. What would it look like to integrate "emotional gear checks" into your team's regular workflow?

Voices from the Fire Service:

"You don't just check your air pack. You check your head, your heart, and your crew. Because no one walks into the fire unready, and no one walks in alone."
- Battalion Chief, Urban Fire Department

Chapter 8 : Kitchen Table Leadership

> *"The strongest leadership doesn't happen in the boardroom. It happens around the kitchen table."*

Every firehouse has one. It might be scratched, mismatched, or built from leftover parts, but the kitchen table is sacred. It's where stories are told, jokes are shared, and truths are spoken. It's where firefighters decompress after calls, welcome the new guy, and grieve the loss of one of their own.

It's not just a place to eat.

It's a place to belong.

In the fire service, the kitchen table is where leadership comes alive not through hierarchy or formal agendas, but through presence. It's where senior members quietly mentor rookies. Where captains listen more than they talk. Where vulnerability isn't seen as weakness, but as evidence of humanity.

And it's where connection is forged not for morale's sake, but for survival.

Now ask yourself:

Where is the kitchen table in nursing?

'In most healthcare settings, we've traded connection for efficiency. Our "break rooms" are storage closets. Our meetings are rushed, virtual, or perfunctory. Our conversations are task-driven, not relationship-centered. In academia, we see faculty passing each other like strangers. In leadership, we often lead through memos instead of moments.

We've lost the table and with it, we've lost something vital.

The Power of Informal Leadership

Leadership isn't a title. And it's not a meeting invite.

It's a moment when someone says, "Tell me what's going on."

It's sharing coffee and really listening.

It's noticing when someone's not okay and sitting down anyway.

The kitchen table in the firehouse reminds us that informal leadership may be the most impactful kind. It's not about control or charisma. It's about consistency, compassion, and conversation.

In nursing, we tend to wait for formal settings to "have the talk." But the most transformative leadership doesn't come from PowerPoint slides, it comes from shared presence. From the leader who lingers after a meeting. Who walks the unit. Who teaches from experience, not ego.

If your leadership doesn't include time at the table with your team, your students, or your peers, you're missing the heartbeat of your influence.

The Table as Equalizer

What's remarkable about the firehouse table is that rank dissolves there.

The new volunteer sits next to the chief. The medic and the firefighter share the same plate. The table doesn't care who makes what or who has what title. It reminds everyone: we are all human, and we all belong.

Nursing desperately needs more of this.

In academia, in hospitals, in national leadership spaces—titles too often separate rather than unite. We hide behind credentials. We assume roles rather than relationships. But people don't follow credentials; they follow character. They follow those who show up, eat with them, and listen to them.

As a leader, ask yourself:

- When was the last time you sat down, informally, with your team, without an agenda?

- Do your staff or students feel safe being themselves around you?

- Is there a space, physical or relational, where your team can be real?

If not, build the table.

It doesn't have to be fancy. It has to be authentic.

Creating "Kitchen Tables" in Nursing Spaces

You can't always replicate the firehouse kitchen table, but you can create its spirit anywhere.

In a hospital:

> Create space for huddles where people can reflect, not just report.
>
> Invite feedback over coffee instead of over forms.

In academia:

> Hold office hours that are for listening, not lecturing.
>
> Host informal lunches where students and faculty can just be.

In leadership:

> Use one-on-ones to connect, not just correct.

Replace "how's the project?" with "how's your heart?"

These are your tables. They don't require a budget. Just your time, your presence, and your willingness to sit with people, not above them.

Leading From the Table

Great leaders don't always lead from the front. Sometimes they lead from the side—at the table—quietly listening, gently guiding, showing others that leadership is a shared meal, not a solo performance.

When leaders show up at the table:

Teams feel seen.

Walls come down.

Trust is built.

And when trust is built, people talk. They share concerns early, before they become crises. They ask for help without shame. They challenge each other with respect. They show up for each other because they remember that someone first showed up for them.

That's what kitchen table leadership does. It doesn't just keep people engaged, it keeps them from leaving.

Leadership Flashpoint: Reflection Prompts

7. Where are your "kitchen tables"? Places for honest, informal connection in your leadership space?

8. How often do you sit down without a formal agenda just to be present with your team?

9. What small rituals can you create to make space for mentorship, vulnerability, or shared humanity?

Voices from the Fire Service:

"Around the table, we're all just people. Titles don't matter. What matters is that you show up with your whole self. That's where the crew becomes a family."
– **Retired Fire Lieutenant, Volunteer Department**

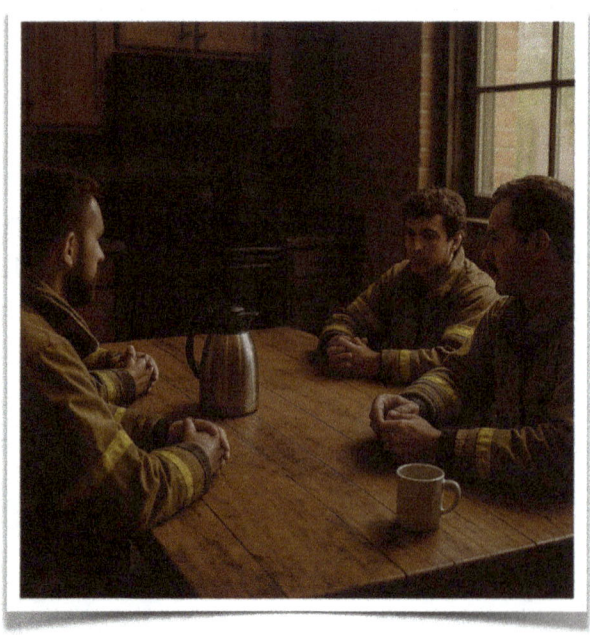

Chapter 9 : Honor the Sacrifice

"In the fire service, when one of us is lost, the bell rings. In nursing, when one of us is lost, the silence is deafening."

Firefighters have a saying: Everyone goes home. And when someone doesn't, when a firefighter is lost in the line of duty, the entire brotherhood responds. Sirens go silent. Flags are lowered. Bagpipes play. Helmets are removed. The bell rings, three sets of five chimes, to honor the fallen. The ritual is solemn, symbolic, and seared into the memory of every firefighter who witnesses it.

Why? Because the sacrifice of one is felt by all. Because no one is forgotten. Because in the fire service, honor is a cornerstone of culture.

Now look at nursing.

When a nurse leaves the profession, broken, burned out, or taken too soon, what do we do?

Often, nothing.

There's no bell.

No tribute.

No pause.

Just a gap on the schedule and a new posting on a job board.

This silence sends a dangerous message: that your presence is only as valuable as your productivity. That your burnout is a personal failure. That your departure is just part of the churn.

Leadership must reject this narrative.

We must honor the sacrifice of nurses, both living and gone, not just through memorials, but through meaning. Through reflection. Through change. Through a collective commitment to never let another colleague disappear unnoticed.

Because when we forget the fallen, we tell the rest: You don't matter either.

The Invisible Losses

Every year, thousands of nurses leave the profession, not due to a lack of skill or passion, but because they feel unseen, unsupported, and unvalued.

- Some leave quietly.

- Some leave abruptly.

- Some stay, but disengage completely, burned out in place, emotionally gone.

These are losses, too. But we don't grieve them. We rationalize them:

"They couldn't handle the pace."

"They were too emotional."

"They weren't a fit for the culture."

But those are just rationalizations. The truth is, we failed them.

- **We failed to listen.**

- **We failed to act.**

- **We failed to honor their contribution before it became a farewell.**

Leadership must begin to view each resignation, each breakdown, each act of moral injury not as an isolated event, but as a red flag. A signal that something in our culture is broken. That something must change.

Recognition is Restoration

In the fire service, honoring sacrifice doesn't just happen at funerals. It happens every day, through rituals, language, memorials, and shared stories. Firefighters wear each other's numbers, tell each other's tales, carry each other's burdens. They don't forget.

This daily remembrance isn't morbid, it's restorative.

It reminds the team: We matter. Our work matters. Our people matter.

Nursing must reclaim this spirit of recognition–not as a reward, but as a restoration.

Leaders, this is your charge:

- **Recognize the emotional toll of the work, openly, consistently, and without shame.**

- **Celebrate contributions, not just outcomes.**

- **Acknowledge grief for patients, for peers, for the parts of ourselves we sometimes lose.**

- **Honor stories, not just stats.**

A profession that does not honor its people cannot sustain itself.

Ritual as Leadership Practice

Rituals bind teams together. They create shared meaning. They tell us who we are and what we value.

The fire service understands this intuitively. From bell ceremonies to helmet retirements to shared meals after tough calls, these moments matter. They bring closure. They bring unity. They keep the humanity in the work.

Nursing has few such rituals left.

What if we brought them back?

A moment of silence at the beginning of faculty meetings for a lost nurse or student. A wall of honor in your clinic or school recognizing nurses who've made a lasting impact. Annual ceremonies not just for awards, but for remembrance and reflection. A monthly time to tell stories, not for evaluation, but for healing.

Leadership isn't just about vision, it's about meaning-making. About creating space for the sacred amidst the daily grind.

Because without meaning, the grind becomes unbearable.

Honoring Ourselves

Let's be honest: sometimes the hardest person to honor is yourself.

As nurse leaders, we often pour into others without pause. We downplay our own struggles. We keep going, even when we're running on empty. But even firefighters have to take a knee, to rehab, to rest.

Nursing leaders must model self-honor:

- Take time to reflect.

- Tell your own story.

- Name your own sacrifices.

- Build in rhythms of renewal, not as exceptions, but as expectations.

You can't pour from an empty cup and you shouldn't have to.

The Bell Must Ring

In the fire service, the bell rings to honor the end of a call and the end of a life. It rings to remind the living that the fallen are not forgotten.

In nursing, we must start ringing our own bells, not just in mourning, but in memory, in mission, and in momentum.

- Let it ring for the nurse who left quietly.

- Let it ring for the one who died too young.

- Let it ring for the burned-out, the disillusioned, the unseen.

- And let it ring for those still here, fighting, leading, hoping.

Let it ring to remind them: You matter. We see you. We will not forget.

Leadership Flashpoint: Reflection Prompts

10. When was the last time you recognized a colleague's emotional or personal sacrifice not just their productivity?

11. What rituals or moments of remembrance does your organization have to honor those who've left, retired, or passed away?

12. How can you integrate daily, weekly, or monthly rhythms of recognition to restore your team's sense of value and purpose?

Voices from the Fire Service:

> **"When the bell rings, it doesn't just mark a loss. It reminds us who we are. And who we never want to lose again."**
> - Chief, Career Fire Department

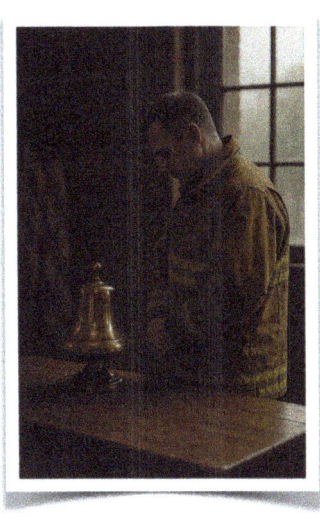

Chapter 10 : The Call We All Heard

"We didn't come to nursing for the pay, the titles, or the policies. We came because we heard the call. Leadership must help us remember it."

There's a moment, quiet and personal, that nearly every nurse can recall. It may have happened in childhood, witnessing a loved one suffer and wanting to help. It may have come later, in a classroom, in combat, in crisis. But for almost all of us, there was a moment, a spark, when we knew this was our path.

That moment wasn't about charting or scheduling. It wasn't about credentials or clinical ladders.

It was about purpose.

And we called it a calling because that's exactly what it felt like.

But somewhere between that first spark and today's burnout statistics, many of us lost the sound of that call. It was drowned out by staff shortages, paperwork, institutional indifference, and endless "initiatives" that failed to ask us who we are or why we do this work.

As nurse leaders, we must become keepers of the call.

Just like fire captains remind their crew why they signed up, to serve, to protect, to run toward the danger, we must remind our nurses, students, faculty, and ourselves:

You didn't come here to survive a shift.

You came here to change lives and to be changed.

The Call Isn't a Myth. It's a Mission.

In the fire service, when a rookie walks through the station doors for the first time, they're often asked, "Why are you here?" It's not a test, it's a grounding question. And when things get hard (and they always do), that same question comes back: Why did you answer the call?

Nursing needs this culture of remembrance.

Our callings are not myths, they are missions.

But a mission requires direction. And leadership must be the compass.

That means:

- Creating time for reflection, even in fast-paced environments.

- Telling stories, not just stats.

- Allowing space for people to reconnect with the why, not just the what.

- Helping teams see the human impact of their work, not just its compliance.

When we forget our calling, the job becomes just that: a job.

And that's when we start to lose each other.

When the Call Becomes a Whisper

For many nurses, the call hasn't disappeared, it's just become a whisper beneath the noise of an overburdened system.

They want to care, but the charting gets in the way. They want to teach, but the bureaucracy suffocates them. They want to lead, but the politics drain their passion. They want to stay, but no one asks them why they're thinking of leaving.

Leadership must listen, not to metrics first, but to meaning.

Ask:

- What drew you to this work?

- What's kept you here?

- What's making it harder to stay?

Don't wait for the exit interview to ask these questions. Ask them now. Ask them often. And don't just collect the answers, act on them.

Because every nurse who leaves without being asked why is a missed opportunity to protect the very heart of our profession.

Reigniting the Call Through Leadership Presence

In the firehouse, senior leaders don't just manage, they mentor. They share war stories. They speak to legacy. They model integrity. They show up not only for duty, but for meaning.

Nursing leadership must do the same.

You can't reignite someone else's call if your own has gone cold.

You must reconnect to your purpose.

You must remember why you answered.

And then you must show up, authentically, vulnerably, consistently, to help others remember too.

That means:

- Telling your story of why you became a nurse, even when it feels raw.

- Speaking openly about the costs of leadership and why they're still worth it.

- Leading not with perfection, but with purpose.

Your presence as a leader is the torch that can relight the flame in others.

The New Generation is Listening

Today's emerging nurses, students, early-career clinicians, new faculty, are watching. They're asking:

Is this profession still worthy of my sacrifice?

Will I find meaning here?

Will I belong?

They're listening for the call, but they're also watching to see if it's still real for you.

So leaders: what are you showing them?

- Are you modeling burnout or boundary setting?

- Are you modeling cynicism or courage?

- Are you showing that this work is still noble even when it's hard?

The call to nursing never promised ease. But it did promise impact, connection, and meaning.

It's time to remind the next generation and ourselves that the call is still ringing.

And that they're not answering it alone.

Leadership Flashpoint: Reflection Prompts

13. What was your original "why" for becoming a nurse or entering this profession? Have you shared it recently?

14. What parts of your work still spark your sense of calling and which parts threaten to extinguish it?

15. How do you help your team reconnect with purpose during times of stress, fatigue, or disillusionment?

Voices from the Fire Service:

"Some days you hear the call loud and clear. Some days it's barely a whisper. But you show up anyway because the fire doesn't wait. And neither do the people who need you."
- Firefighter and Veteran Medic

Chapter 11 : Lighting the Next Torch

"Every torch that burns brightly was lit by another."

There's a moment in every firefighter's journey when the shift from student to steward takes place. You're no longer just learning the ropes; you're showing others how to tie them. You're no longer asking the questions; you're answering them. You're not just carrying the torch; you're preparing to pass it on.

And that moment, when recognized and honored, becomes one of the most sacred transitions in the fire service.

Nursing, too, is a profession of lineage, of stories, skills, and strength passed from one generation to the next. But in our haste to fill positions and meet benchmarks, we often miss the power of this passing of the torch. We forget that leadership isn't just about what you build; it's about who you build up.

The truth is, we will all leave the profession someday.

The question is:

Will we leave it better than we found it?

Will we leave it brighter for those who follow?

Mentorship Is a Moral Obligation

In the firehouse, mentorship isn't an optional program; it's a duty. Veterans take rookies under their wing not because they have time, but because they were once rookies too. And someone did the same for them.

It's not formalized. It's not forced. It's cultural.

In nursing, mentorship is often formalized into checklists and occasional meetings. But the real mentorship, the kind that changes lives, happens in the margins: in the hallway after a hard shift, over coffee after a failed grant, in the gentle correction offered without shame.

Leadership must elevate mentorship from an HR initiative to a sacred leadership practice.

Mentorship Is:

- Investing time when no one's watching.

- Offering perspective without superiority.

- Helping others find their voice, their confidence, their calling.

- And perhaps most importantly, mentorship is about believing in someone before they believe in themselves.

Your Legacy Is Not Your Résumé

There's nothing wrong with accomplishments. But your titles, your publications, your accolades–they are not your legacy.

Your legacy is in:

- The student who stayed because of your encouragement.

- The nurse who speaks up now because you showed her how.

- The leader who leads with integrity because they watched you do it.

- The person who was about to quit but saw something in you that gave them hope.

The fire service understands this. Retirements are emotional, not because someone's leaving a position, but because someone's leaving a mark.

Nursing must rediscover this kind of legacy.

Leadership is not about being the star of the story. It's about multiplying impact through others.

The Torch is Lit Through Trust

You cannot pass a torch you haven't lit.

If you want to develop the next generation of nurse leaders, educators, and innovators, you have to:

Trust them.

Challenge them.

Empower them.

Stop hoarding leadership out of fear. Stop gatekeeping because "they're not ready." No one was ready the first time. Someone made them ready by walking alongside them.

Let go of perfection. Let go of ego. Let go of legacy as personal achievement.

The brightest fire comes from shared flame.

And when you hand the torch over, do it with joy, not resentment. The next generation doesn't threaten your worth; they extend it.

Creating a Culture of Continuity

Firehouses don't reinvent the culture with every new hire. They pass it on. Through rituals. Through stories. Through expectations. Through example.

Nursing must do the same.

Leaders should ask:

- What are we passing on?

- What values are we reinforcing in the way we treat new grads, new faculty, or emerging leaders?

- What behaviors are we tolerating that erode our culture?

- What traditions should we preserve–and what outdated norms must we release?

Culture isn't written; it's witnessed. It's carried in people, not policy.

You are writing your leadership legacy right now, not in what you do, but in who you lift.

The Future Is Watching

Never forget this: Someone is watching you. Right now. A student. A new hire. A future leader who doesn't yet know their own potential.

They are watching to see:

- How you respond when things go wrong.

- How you treat people who can't offer you anything.

- How you lead when no one is looking.

They are watching because they are trying to figure out what's possible.

So show them.

Show them how to lead with heart.

Show them how to stand in fire and still stay human.

Show them how to light the next torch, so that when your light dims, theirs burns even brighter.

Leadership Flashpoint: Reflection Prompts

16. Who mentored you and how are you honoring their legacy in your leadership?

17. Who in your orbit are you currently mentoring or investing in?

18. What would it look like to lead in a way that multiplies, rather than centralizes, your impact?

Voices from the Fire Service:

"The best leaders don't just train the next crew. They build them, believe in them, and then step back to watch them shine."

- Retired Fire Chief, State Fire Academy

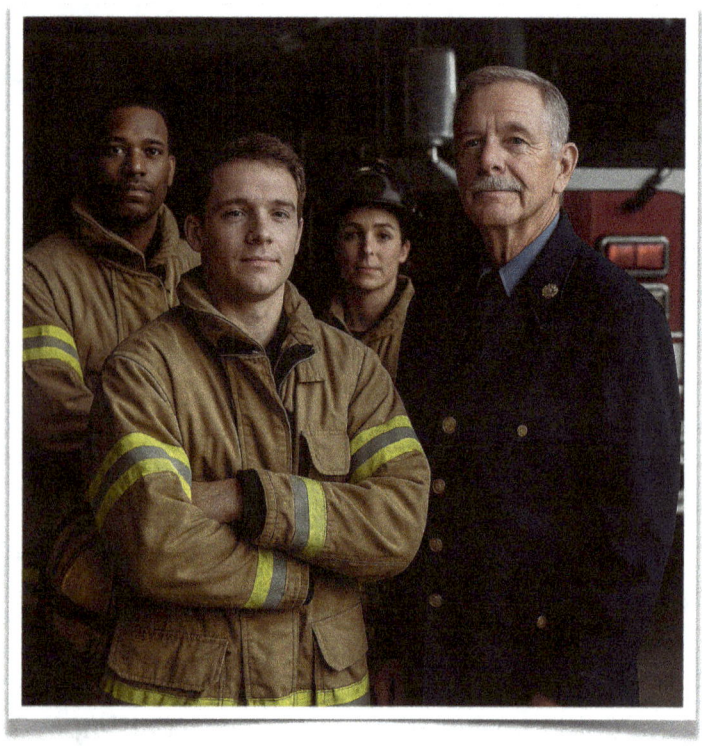

Chapter 12 : A Profession Worth Saving

"You don't run into a burning building unless what's inside is worth saving. The same is true for nursing."

Firefighters don't enter flames for the adrenaline. They do it for the people trapped inside, the mother, the child, the brother, the stranger. They go in because they believe what's at risk is worth it. That's what makes them brave. That's what makes them run toward danger when others are running away.

Nursing is on fire.

Burnout is rising.

Moral injury is deepening.

Disconnection is spreading.

And people, good people, are leaving.

But we haven't lost the profession. We've lost the connection to its soul.

And if we believe this profession is worth saving and it is, then leaders must be the ones to run back in. Not alone. Not recklessly. But together, strategically, with clarity and conviction, ready to rebuild what has been damaged, and reignite what has been dimmed.

Because this isn't just a profession. This is a calling. A purpose. A legacy.

The Fire is Real and So Is the Fight

Nursing is suffering not just from external pressures, but from internal silence.

We've accepted burnout as a badge of honor.

We've normalized disconnection as a part of the job.

We've let fear drive policy and let policy drive people away.

But what if we stopped managing the crisis and started leading through it?

In the fire service, they don't enter a blaze without a plan, without backup, or without someone watching their six. They train, they trust, and they talk. Constantly.

Nursing must do the same:

- Train our leaders not just in systems, but in human connection.

- Build teams that trust not just comply.

- Open the doors to honest, courageous dialogue about what we're facing.

We don't save this profession through metrics.
We save it through meaning.

You Are the First-In Team

In fire terminology, the first-in team is the one that gets there first, that takes initial command, that faces the unknown before anyone else arrives.

If you're reading this, you are part of that first-in team for a new era of nursing.

You're the one kicking in the door to make room for others to breathe.

You're leading the charge not because it's easy, but because you heard the call. And you chose to answer it.

You don't have to do it alone. But you do have to go first:

- First to name the burnout.

- First to rebuild connection.

- First to mentor with authenticity.

- First to lead from the table, not the tower.

- First to say: "I remember why I started. And I still believe."

What We're Saving

We're not just saving roles or schedules.

We're saving the profession that:

- Sat at thousands of bedsides in the darkest moments of people's lives.

- Advocated for equity when others stayed silent.

- Raised up leaders who didn't just manage systems but healed them.

- Inspired young people to enter a field that promises more than a paycheck; it promises purpose.

We're saving the soul of a profession that has never just been about care tasks or clinical notes.

We're saving a profession built on:

> **Humanity**
>
> **Connection**
>
> **Service**
>
> **Sacrifice**

A profession that, like the fire service, is rooted in altruism, brotherhood, courage, and relentless hope.

The Rebuild Begins With You

Fire scenes eventually go cold. And when they do, the crews begin the work of rebuilding. They clear the debris. They secure the structure. They support the victims. And then they return home not just to rest, but to prepare for the next call.

Nursing is in that rebuilding phase.

Yes, we're tired. But we're not done. Yes, we've lost people. But not our why. Yes, we've been burned. But the fire has also revealed what must change.

As a leader, you are the architect of that rebuild.

And the blueprint is simple:

> **Lead with presence.**
> **Connect before you correct.**
> **Build belonging as your strategy.**
> **Honor the sacrifice.**
> **Pass the torch.**
> **Light the way.**

Because this isn't just a profession worth working in.
This is a profession worth saving.

Leadership Flashpoint: Final Reflection Prompts

19. What will you do in the next 30 days to re-establish deeper connection with your team?

20. Who in your organization needs to be seen, heard, or supported right now?

21. What legacy are you actively building and who are you building it for?

Voices from the Fire Service:

"We don't run into the fire for the glory. We do it because someone has to go first. Someone has to believe that what's inside is still worth it. And someone has to carry the others back out."
- Battalion Chief, Retired

Epilogue: The Bell Tolls Once More

One day, the bell will ring for each of us. Not just in death, but in departure, from a role, from a career, from the profession. When it does, may we leave knowing that we lit more torches than we burned out. That we built a stronger house than we inherited. And that we answered the call not just once, but every time it mattered.

Because that's what real leadership does.

>It shows up.

>It connects.

>It serves.

>And it saves.

Final Words from the Fire Service

"When the last bell rings for you, it won't matter how many fires you fought or how many shifts you worked. What will matter is who's still standing because you stood for them, who's carrying the torch you lit, and how many knew they were never in the fight alone."
- Retired Fire Chief, 35 Years of Service

In Memoriam

Dr. Jiayun Xu (1987-2025)

> *"In the fire service, when one of us is lost, the bell rings. In nursing, when one of us is lost, the silence is deafening."*

On August 2, 2025, we lost our friend and colleague, **Dr. Jiayun Xu,** a brilliant nurse scientist, a devoted partner and mother, and a fierce advocate for people and families facing serious illness. She died peacefully after a brief, courageous 29-day fight with stage IV colon cancer. She was 37.

Born in Wuxi, China, Jiayun's journey carried her across disciplines and institutions, but always toward the same North Star: easing suffering and restoring dignity at life's most vulnerable edges. At Oregon Health & Science University, she served as a nurse scientist with the Parkinson's Disease and Movement Disorders team, advancing quality improvement and research to better the lives of patients and families navigating neurodegenerative disease. Before that, she served on the faculty at Purdue University's School of Nursing, where her work in **advance care planning** helped families prepare for difficult decisions long before crisis arrived.

Jiayun's scholarship lived where **science meets humanity**. She examined how caregivers communicate with clinicians in home hospice, how burden erodes wellbeing, and how nurses can lead palliative care forward. Her publications and collaborations, in palliative, hospice, and caregiver research, shaped practice and invited nurses to claim their rightful place at the center of serious-illness care.

Jiayun refused that silence in her work; she insisted that we **name** the toll, **see** the person, and **plan** with compassion. To honor her is to refuse the quiet acceptance of burnout, moral injury, and invisible grief in our ranks. It is to build rituals of remembrance and rhythms of restoration into the way we lead.

So we ring the bell here, for the scientist who made care more human, for the colleague whose questions were as gentle as they were incisive, for the friend whose laughter cut through long days. We ring it for the mother and partner whose love steadied a family; for the mentor who opened doors; for the nurse who taught us that preparing families for hard moments is itself an act of hope.

The bell must ring, in mourning, in memory, and in momentum. Let it ring for Jiayun, and let its echo be our charge:

- to tell the stories behind the statistics;
- to build rituals that recognize the emotional labor of nursing;

- to design systems that prevent the next preventable loss.

Five-five-five for Dr. Jiayun Xu. We will not forget.

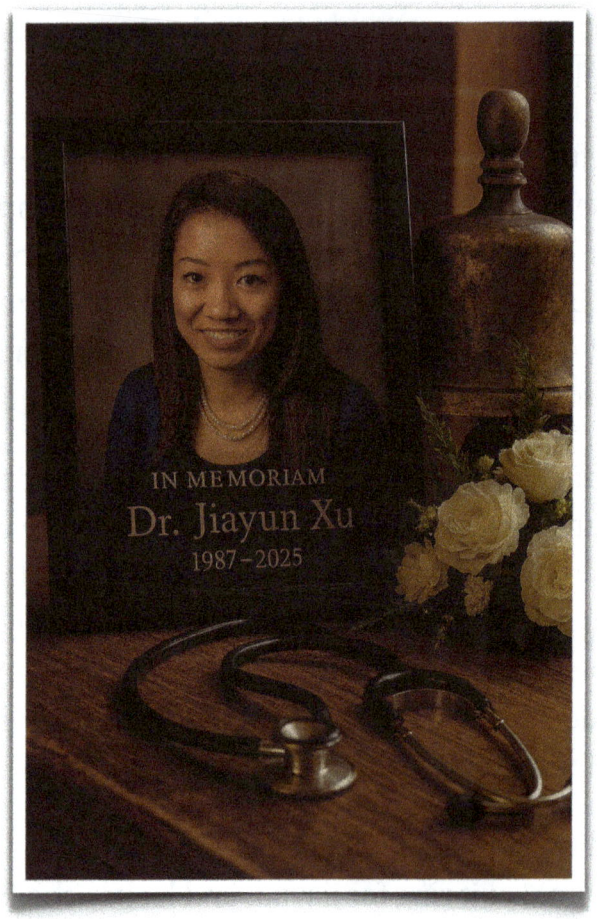

Workbook

Chapter 1 : Welcome to the Firehouse

Creating a Culture of Welcome

FIREHOUSE LEADERSHIP TACTIC

Start every team gathering with a moment of presence. Make space for names, stories, and shared values.

Reflection Prompt

What can you do to create a more welcoming environment for your team or colleagues?

Journal Reflection

Describe a time you felt welcomed. How can you recreate that for others?

SMART Goal Examples

- Start a weekly welcome huddle for all staff
- Create a buddy system for new hires
- Share a weekly 'story of connection' at staff meetings

Potential Barriers

- Lack of time or staff buy-in

- High turnover disrupting continuity
- Overloaded orientation processes

Support Resources

- Peer mentors
- Onboarding materials

Target Completion Date

Progress Notes

Chapter 2 : The Brotherhood is Built, Not Assigned

Building Brotherhood Through Trust

FIREHOUSE LEADERSHIP TACTIC

Don't assume trust, build it. Invest in rituals, shared meals, and honest conversations with your crew.

Reflection Prompt

How can you intentionally build trust and mutual respect among your peers?

Journal Reflection

When did you feel a deep sense of trust in a team? What built it?

SMART Goal Examples

- Initiate trust-building discussions with your team
- Recognize peer-to-peer support in team emails
- Conduct crew evaluations focused on teamwork

Potential Barriers

- History of mistrust or lack of transparency
- Fear of vulnerability in team settings
- Poor modeling from leadership

Support Resources

- Team-building activities
- Leadership support

Target Completion Date

Progress Notes

Chapter 3 : Brotherhood Is Inclusive, Not Exclusive

Inclusive Brotherhood and Belonging

FIREHOUSE LEADERSHIP TACTIC

Make inclusion a ritual. Pair new hires with diverse mentors and share origin stories often.

Reflection Prompt

What actions can you take to ensure inclusivity and solidarity in your workplace?

Journal Reflection

Have you ever felt excluded? How did it affect you?

SMART Goal Examples

- Facilitate a workshop on inclusive practices.
- Develop a DEI mentorship matching system.
- Host storytelling circles featuring underrepresented individuals.

Potential Barriers

- Institutional resistance to change.
- Lack of representation at leadership levels.
- Unspoken micro-aggressions or exclusion.

Support Resources

- DEI committee.
- Inclusive training workshops.

Target Completion Date

Progress Notes

Chapter 4: Who Answers the Alarm?

Hearing the Alarms Around You

FIREHOUSE LEADERSHIP TACTIC

Do a weekly roll call, not just who's here, but who seems distant. Reach out before the silence grows.

Reflection Prompt

Whose 'alarm' have you missed lately, and how can you show up for them moving forward?

Journal Reflection

Think of someone who may be struggling. How can you support them?

SMART Goal Examples

- Schedule biweekly wellness check-ins with staff.
- Create an anonymous 'call for help' suggestion box.
- Develop a quiet recovery space on the unit.

Potential Barriers

- Emotional burnout masking distress.
- Fear of judgment if struggling.
- Limited emotional support systems.

Support Resources

- Employee assistance programs.
- Peer check-ins.

Target Completion Date

Progress Notes

Chapter 5: Accountability at the Fire Scene

Accountability as Protection

FIREHOUSE LEADERSHIP TACTIC

Use the 'accountability officer' model, assign someone to track not just tasks but people's well-being.

Reflection Prompt

How do you model accountability, and what systems can you implement to improve it?

Journal Reflection

Write about a moment when accountability protected someone. How can you replicate that?

SMART Goal Examples

- Implement a weekly team accountability huddle
- Assign rotating 'team safety lead' roles
- Launch an end-of-project team debriefing form

Potential Barriers

- Past negative experiences with accountability
- Fear of punishment or blame
- Ambiguous reporting structure

Support Resources

- Templates for team debriefs
- Facilitation guides

Target Completion Date

Progress Notes

Chapter 6: Everyone Has a Role on the Rig

Role Clarity and Team Cohesion

FIREHOUSE LEADERSHIP TACTIC

Lead a 'rig check' for your team—clarify each person's role and affirm how their work impacts others.

Reflection Prompt

Are your team members clear about their roles? How can you help enhance clarity and respect?

Journal Reflection

Reflect on how you see your role in the team. Are you clear and confident?

SMART Goal Examples

- Clarify and publish job roles for your unit
- Hold team meetings to realign tasks to roles
- Celebrate each member's contributions monthly

Potential Barriers

- Role overlap and unclear job descriptions
- Perfectionism and micromanagement tendencies
- Overworked team members

Support Resources

- Job descriptions
- Coaching for team leads

Target Completion Date

Progress Notes

Chapter 7: Checking Your Gear

Emotional Readiness and Gear Checks

FIREHOUSE LEADERSHIP TACTIC

Begin meetings with emotional check-ins. Normalize the question: 'How's your head? How's your heart?'

Reflection Prompt

What emotional or mental 'gear' do you need to check in with more consistently?

Journal Reflection

How are you really feeling today? What are you holding in?

SMART Goal Examples

- Begin daily emotional readiness check-ins
- Encourage 10-minute journaling before shifts
- Provide access to mental health self-assessment tools

Potential Barriers

- Cultural stigma around mental health
- Lack of time for self-assessment
- Poor boundary-setting habits

Support Resources

- Mindfulness apps
- Resilience training

Target Completion Date

Progress Notes

Chapter 8: Kitchen Table Leadership

Leading from the Kitchen Table

FIREHOUSE LEADERSHIP TACTIC

Host a no-agenda lunch monthly. Sit side by side. Share something personal before discussing work.

Reflection Prompt

Where is your 'kitchen table' and how can you create more informal connection opportunities?

Journal Reflection

What is a conversation you've had that made you feel truly heard?

SMART Goal Examples

- Host a biweekly coffee roundtable with your team
- Use 'walk-and-talks' for informal feedback.
- Create a question jar for honest, anonymous input.

Potential Barriers

- Lack of physical space for informal gatherings.
- Focus on tasks over relationships.
- Virtual or siloed teams.

Support Resources

- Time allocation.
- Coffee chats.
- Check-in circles.

Target Completion Date

Progress Notes

Chapter 9: Honor the Sacrifice

Honoring the Sacrifice of Nurses

FIREHOUSE LEADERSHIP TACTIC

Establish a ritual of remembrance, whether a photo wall, bell ringing, or moment of silence monthly.

Reflection Prompt

How do you currently honor the sacrifices of your colleagues, and what new rituals could you begin?

Journal Reflection

Describe a loss or departure that stuck with you. How was it handled?

SMART Goal Examples

- Develop a remembrance board for former colleagues.
- Celebrate with personal stories.
- Hold a quarterly appreciation huddle.

Potential Barriers

- Fast-paced environments that don't allow pausing.
- Leadership discomfort with emotion.
- Disconnection from mission.

Support Resources

- Inclusion champions.
- Cultural assessments.

Target Completion Date

Progress Notes

Chapter 10: The Call We All Heard

Reconnecting to Your Why

FIREHOUSE LEADERSHIP TACTIC

Have everyone write and share their 'call to nursing' story. Reignite their reason to stay.

Reflection Prompt

> *What sparked your original passion for nursing, and how can you reignite it today?*

Journal Reflection

> *What inspired you to enter nursing? Write about that spark.*

SMART Goal Examples

- Share your 'call to nursing' story during orientation
- Ask your team to write and post their own whys
- Build an annual "Why I Stay" campaign

Potential Barriers

- Institutional focus on output over meaning
- Infrequent reflection opportunities
- Fear of appearing 'soft'

Support Resources

- Storytelling circles
- reflective writing sessions

Target Completion Date

Progress Notes

Chapter 11: Lighting the Next Torch

Mentorship and Torch-Lighting

FIREHOUSE LEADERSHIP TACTIC

Pick one person to mentor, and make the investment visible. Torch lighting is both act and ritual.

Reflection Prompt

> *Who are you mentoring, and how are you actively investing in the next generation?*

Journal Reflection

> *Who saw potential in you before you saw it in yourself?*

SMART Goal Examples

- Mentor one student or staff member per year
- Schedule monthly growth check-ins
- Develop a leadership toolkit for emerging leaders

Potential Barriers

- No formal mentorship program
- Lack of leadership development pathways
- Imposter syndrome or self-doubt

Support Resources

- Mentor training guides
- scheduled check-ins

Target Completion Date

Progress Notes

Chapter 12: A Profession Worth Saving

Saving the Soul of the Profession

FIREHOUSE LEADERSHIP TACTIC

Declare what's worth saving aloud. Invite others to share what nursing means to them–and why it's sacred.

Reflection Prompt

What part of nursing do you believe is worth saving, and what actions will you take to protect it?

Journal Reflection

Why do you believe nursing is worth fighting for?

SMART Goal Examples

- Lead a town hall on the future of nursing
- Partner with others to host a values-based retreat
- Write a vision letter to your future nursing self

Potential Barriers

- Resistance to systemic change
- Cynicism among burned-out staff
- Competing organizational priorities

Support Resources

- Policy advocacy guides
- Leadership coaching

Target Completion Date

Progress Notes

www.ingramcontent.com/pod-product-compliance
Lightning Source LLC
Chambersburg PA
CBHW072202160426
43197CB00012B/2488

www.ingramcontent.com/pod-product-compliance
Lightning Source LLC
Chambersburg PA
CBHW072202160426
43197CB00012B/2488